THIS PLANNER
BELONGS TO

○ ○

Index

Sutras of Pantanjali "The physical
2 Treading the Path postures should be
steady and comfortable.

Strength

21.04.21

1

1 Cat, 2 Balancing Table
3 Tiger 5 Striking
Cobra, 6 + 7 Palm
tree + swaying palm
8 Standing Yoga Seal

✓

Yoga nidra
"running
water"

9 Warrior 1   10 Warrior II
19 Chair   18 Tree
20 Standing forward
bend
37 Extended Child's pose
39 Half boat
30 Bridge

30   Bridge
45 Half. spinal
        twist
47 Savasana
50 Ocean breathing

☆☆☆☆☆

Introduction

Cat + cow - balancing
warm up

Warm up

Cat/cow   balancing table

Main body

Salute to the
moon / Salute to
the sun.

Cool down

Date

28. 04. 21

No of attendees

1

Private Class

✓

Notes

Yoga
nidra

side to side
running
water - stream
waterfall.

Feedback

☆☆☆☆☆

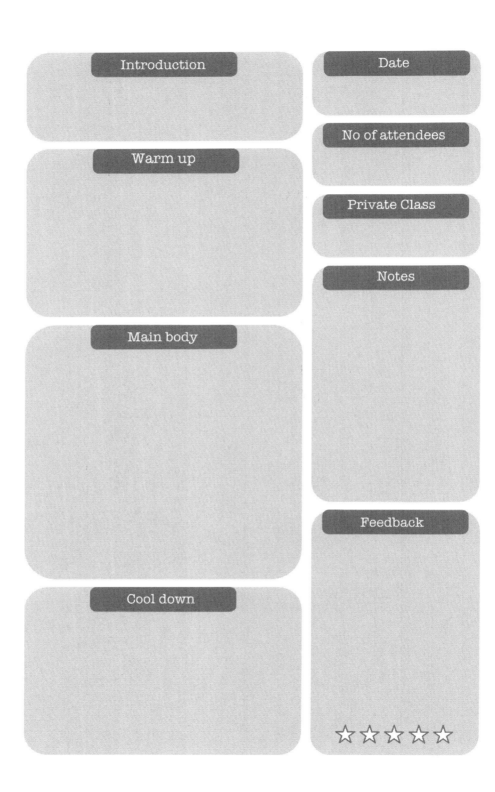

Introduction

Date

Warm up

No of attendees

Private Class

Main body

Notes

Feedback

Cool down

☆☆☆☆☆

Introduction

Date

Warm up

No of attendees

Private Class

Notes

Main body

Feedback

Cool down

☆ ☆ ☆ ☆ ☆

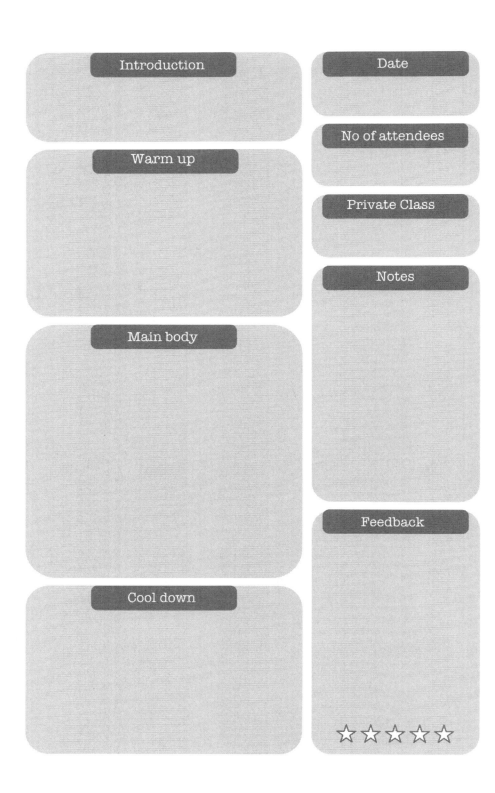

Introduction

Warm up

Main body

Cool down

Date

No of attendees

Private Class

Notes

Feedback

☆☆☆☆☆

Introduction

Date

Warm up

No of attendees

Private Class

Main body

Notes

Feedback

Cool down

☆ ☆ ☆ ☆ ☆

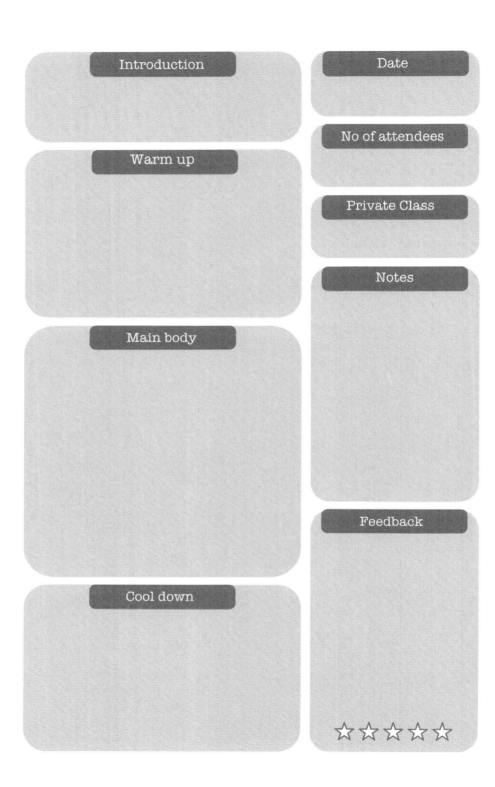

Introduction

Date

Warm up

No of attendees

Private Class

Main body

Notes

Cool down

Feedback

☆☆☆☆☆

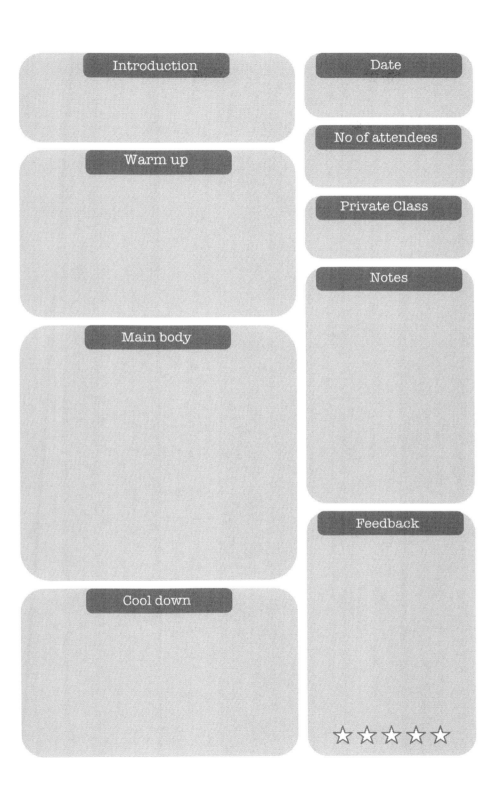

Introduction

Date

Warm up

No of attendees

Private Class

Notes

Main body

Feedback

Cool down

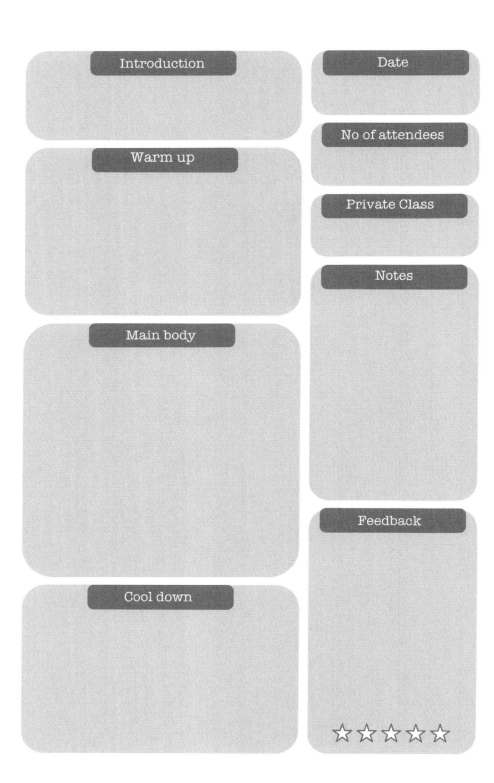

Introduction

Date

Warm up

No of attendees

Private Class

Main body

Notes

Cool down

Feedback

☆☆☆☆☆

Introduction

Date

Warm up

No of attendees

Private Class

Main body

Notes

Feedback

Cool down

☆ ☆ ☆ ☆ ☆

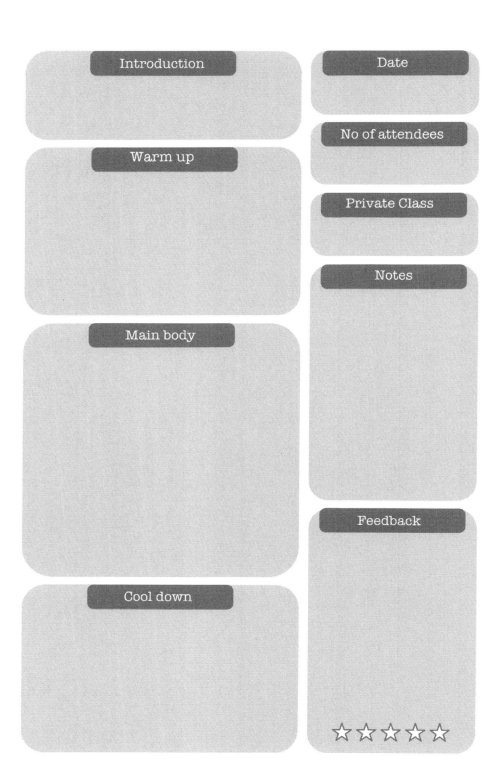

Introduction

Date

Warm up

No of attendees

Private Class

Notes

Main body

Feedback

Cool down

☆☆☆☆☆

Introduction

Warm up

Main body

Cool down

Date

No of attendees

Private Class

Notes

Feedback

☆ ☆ ☆ ☆ ☆

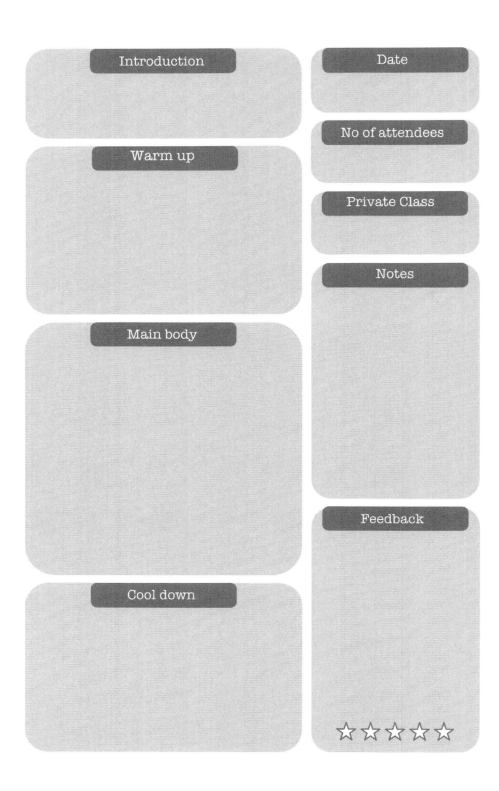

Introduction

Warm up

Main body

Cool down

Date

No of attendees

Private Class

Notes

Feedback

☆☆☆☆☆

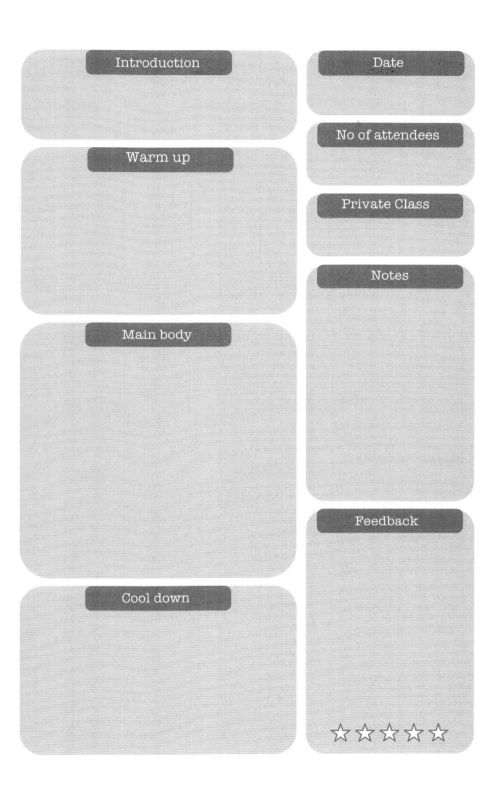

Introduction

Date

Warm up

No of attendees

Private Class

Main body

Notes

Cool down

Feedback

☆☆☆☆☆

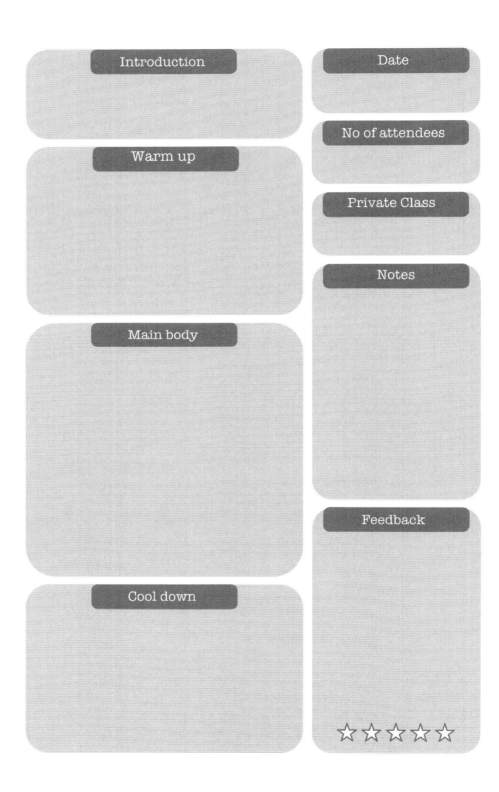

Introduction

Warm up

Main body

Cool down

Date

No of attendees

Private Class

Notes

Feedback

☆ ☆ ☆ ☆ ☆

Introduction

Date

Warm up

No of attendees

Private Class

Notes

Main body

Feedback

Cool down

☆ ☆ ☆ ☆ ☆

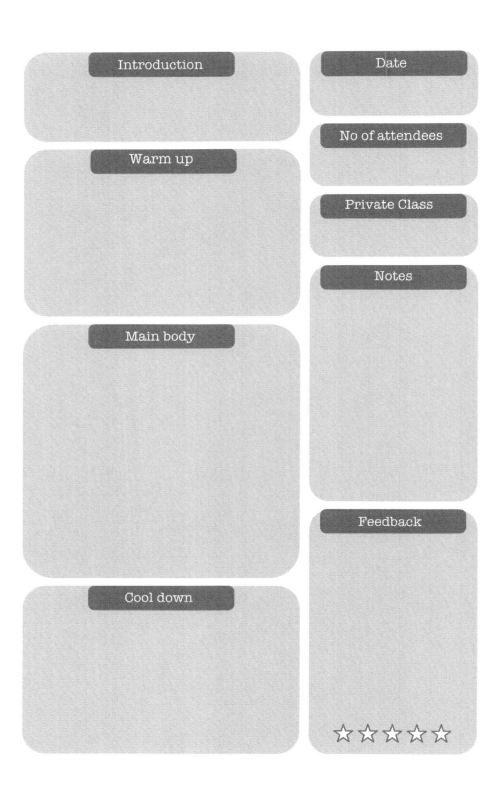

Introduction

Date

Warm up

No of attendees

Private Class

Notes

Main body

Cool down

Feedback

☆☆☆☆☆

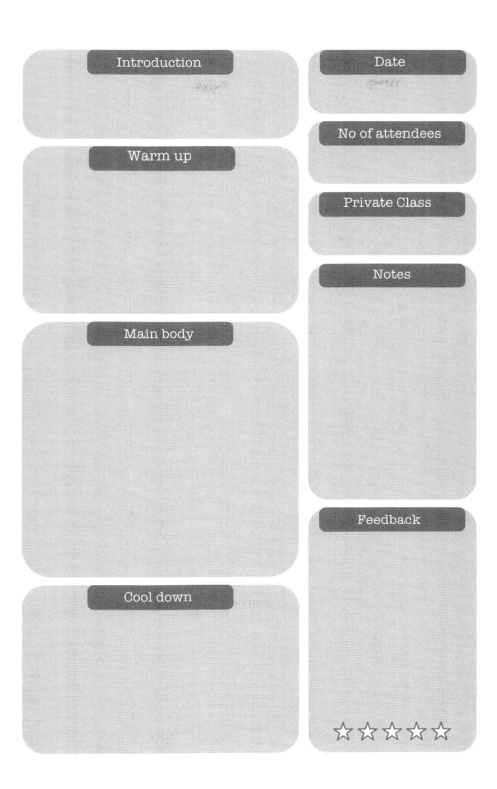

Introduction

Date

No of attendees

Warm up

Private Class

Notes

Main body

Feedback

Cool down

☆☆☆☆☆

Introduction

Warm up

Main body

Cool down

Date

No of attendees

Private Class

Notes

Feedback

☆ ☆ ☆ ☆ ☆

Introduction

Date

No of attendees

Warm up

Private Class

Notes

Main body

Cool down

Feedback

☆ ☆ ☆ ☆ ☆

Introduction

Warm up

Main body

Cool down

Date

No of attendees

Private Class

Notes

Feedback

☆ ☆ ☆ ☆ ☆

Introduction

Date

Warm up

No of attendees

Private Class

Main body

Notes

Feedback

Cool down

☆☆☆☆☆

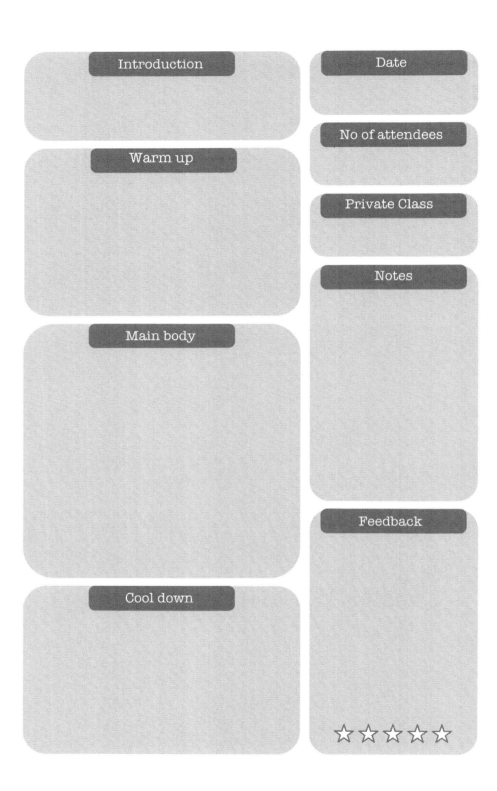

Introduction

Date

Warm up

No of attendees

Private Class

Main body

Notes

Cool down

Feedback

☆☆☆☆☆

Introduction

Date

Warm up

No of attendees

Private Class

Notes

Main body

Cool down

Feedback

☆ ☆ ☆ ☆ ☆

Introduction

Warm up

Main body

Cool down

Date

No of attendees

Private Class

Notes

Feedback

☆☆☆☆☆

Introduction

Date

Warm up

No of attendees

Private Class

Main body

Notes

Feedback

Cool down

☆ ☆ ☆ ☆ ☆

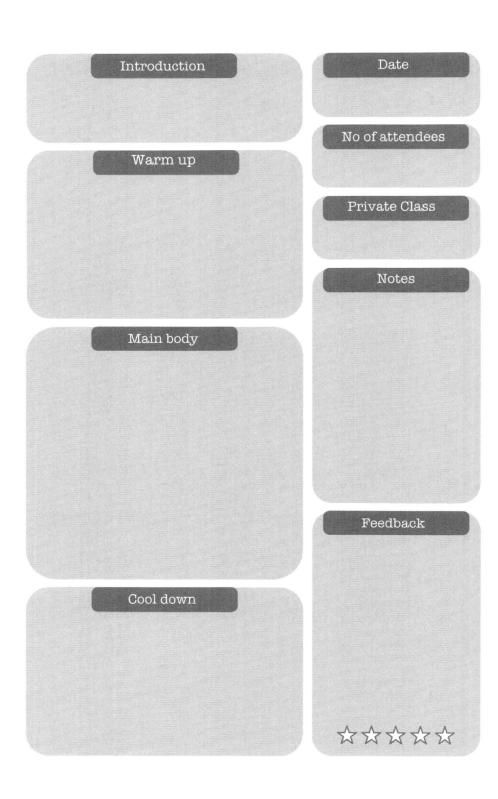

Introduction

Date

Warm up

No of attendees

Private Class

Notes

Main body

Feedback

Cool down

☆☆☆☆☆

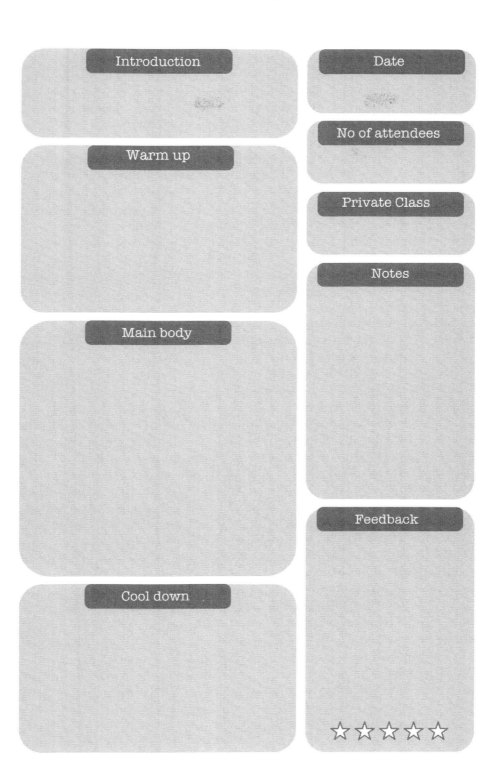

Introduction

Date

No of attendees

Warm up

Private Class

Main body

Notes

Cool down

Feedback

☆☆☆☆☆

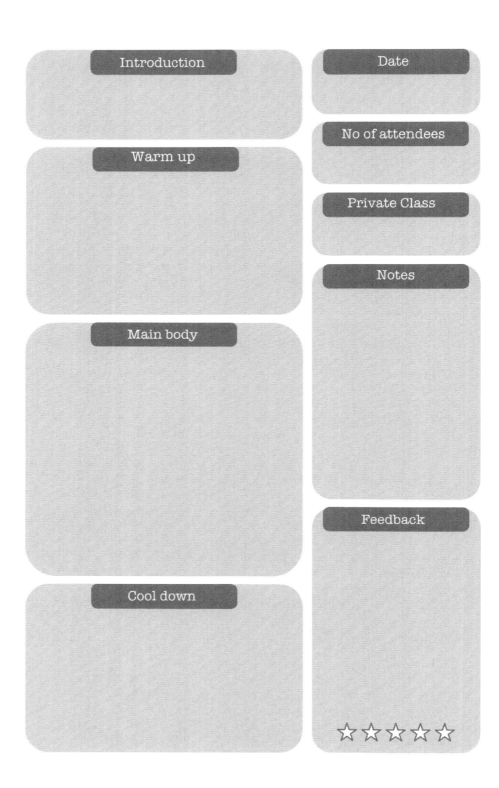

Introduction

Date

Warm up

No of attendees

Private Class

Notes

Main body

Feedback

Cool down

☆☆☆☆☆

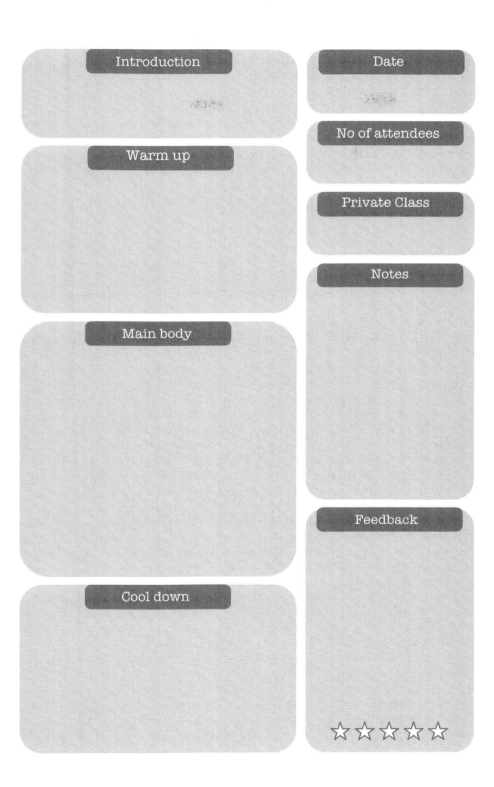

Introduction

Date

Warm up

No of attendees

Private Class

Notes

Main body

Cool down

Feedback

☆☆☆☆☆

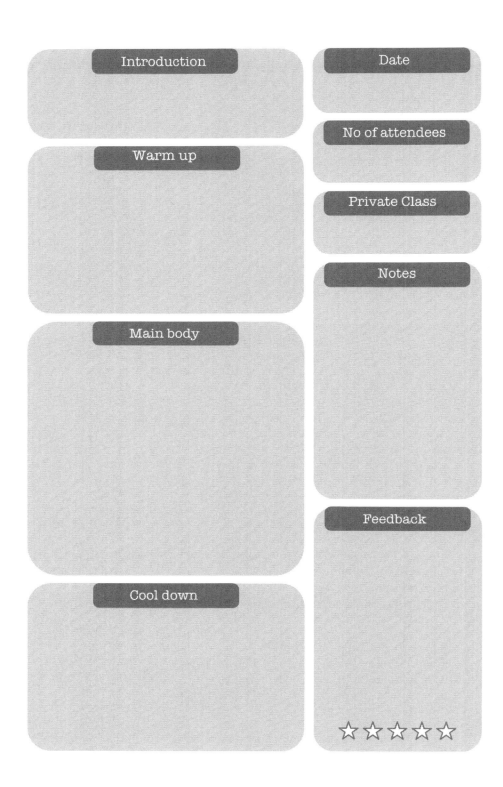

Introduction

Date

Warm up

No of attendees

Private Class

Notes

Main body

Feedback

Cool down

☆☆☆☆☆

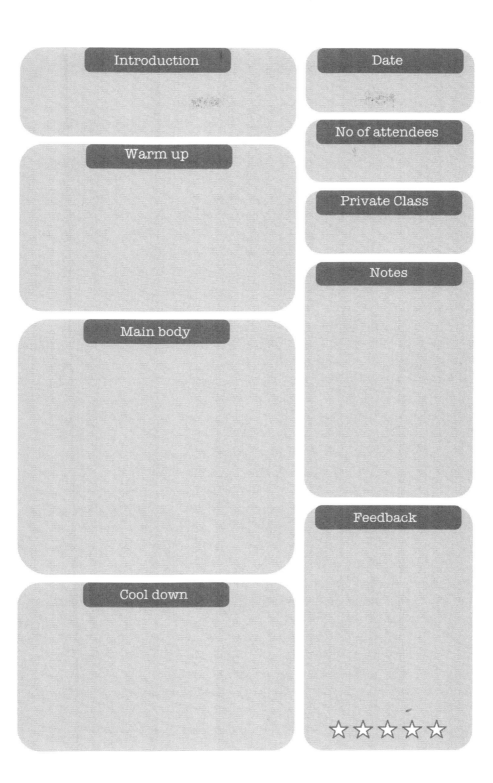

Introduction

Date

Warm up

No of attendees

Private Class

Notes

Main body

Feedback

Cool down

☆☆☆☆☆

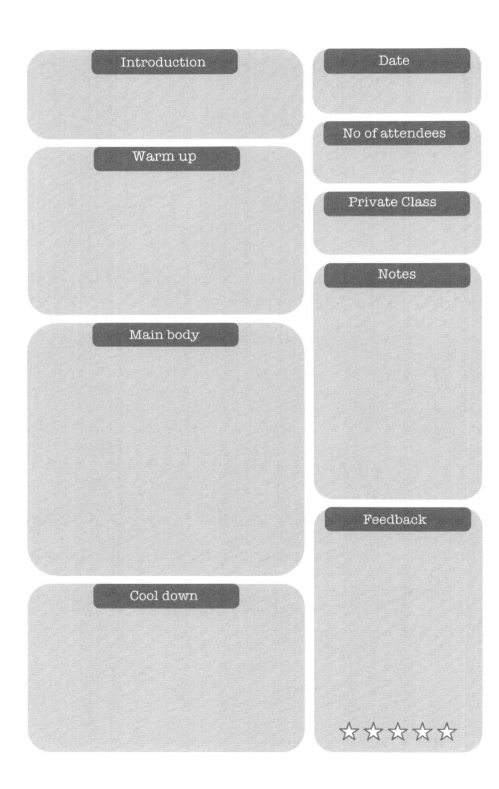

Introduction

Date

No of attendees

Private Class

Warm up

Notes

Main body

Feedback

Cool down

☆☆☆☆☆

Introduction

Date

Warm up

No of attendees

Private Class

Notes

Main body

Feedback

Cool down

☆ ☆ ☆ ☆ ☆

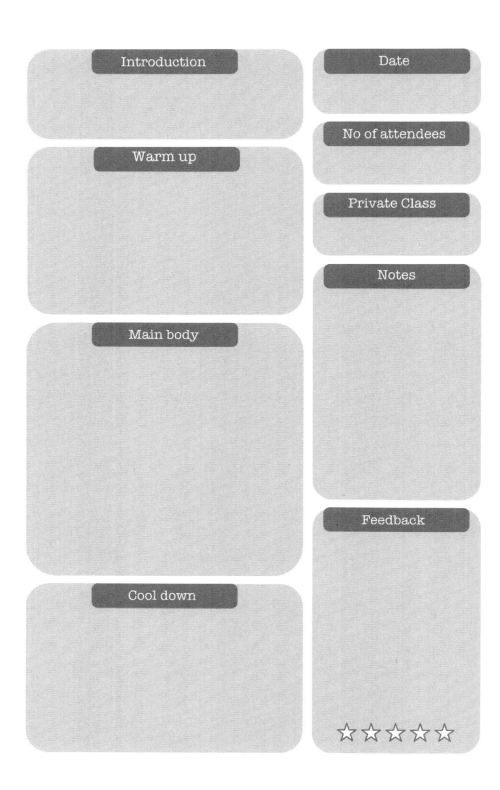

Introduction

Date

Warm up

No of attendees

Private Class

Main body

Notes

Cool down

Feedback

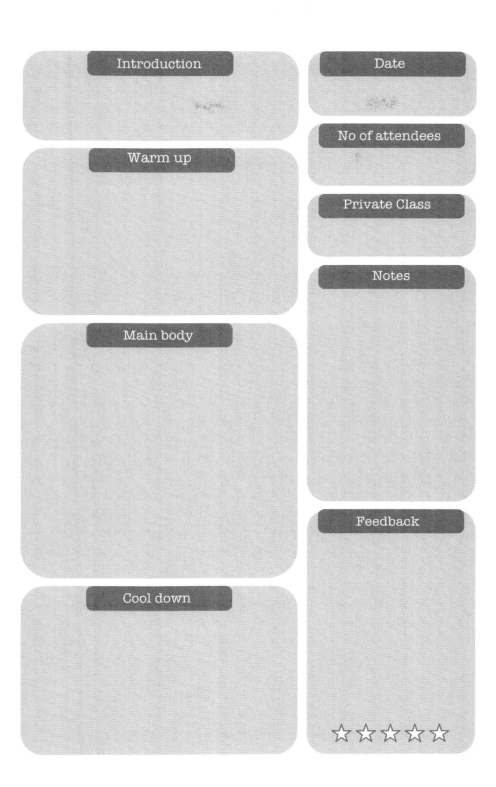

Introduction

Date

No of attendees

Warm up

Private Class

Notes

Main body

Feedback

Cool down

☆☆☆☆☆

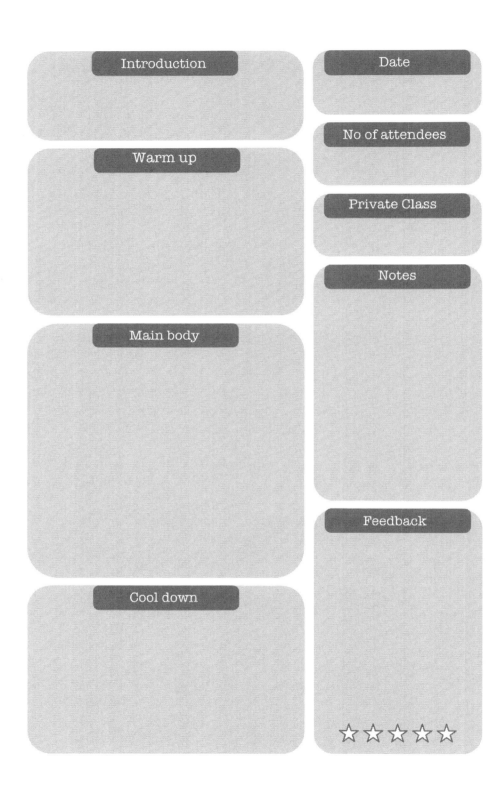

Introduction

Date

Warm up

No of attendees

Private Class

Main body

Notes

Feedback

Cool down

☆☆☆☆☆

Introduction

Date

No of attendees

Warm up

Private Class

Notes

Main body

Cool down

Feedback

☆☆☆☆☆

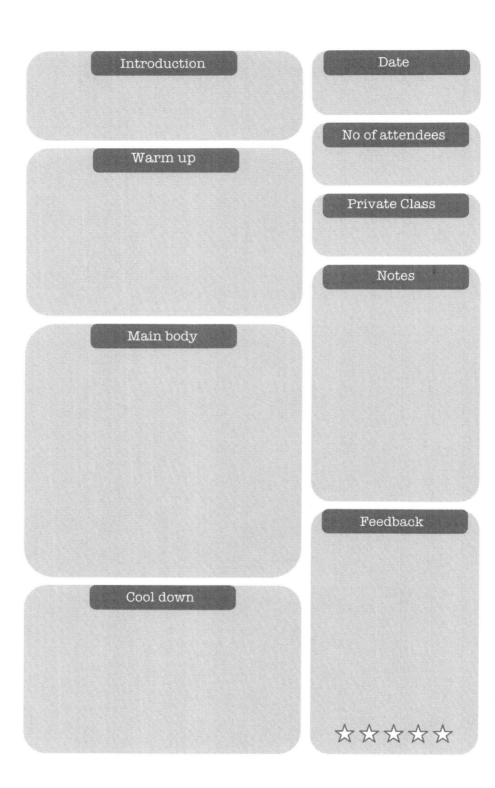

Introduction

Date

Warm up

No of attendees

Private Class

Main body

Notes

Cool down

Feedback

☆☆☆☆☆

Introduction

Date

No of attendees

Warm up

Private Class

Notes

Main body

Feedback

Cool down

☆ ☆ ☆ ☆ ☆

Introduction

Date

No of attendees

Warm up

Private Class

Main body

Notes

Cool down

Feedback

☆ ☆ ☆ ☆ ☆

Introduction

Date

Warm up

No of attendees

Private Class

Main body

Notes

Cool down

Feedback

☆ ☆ ☆ ☆ ☆

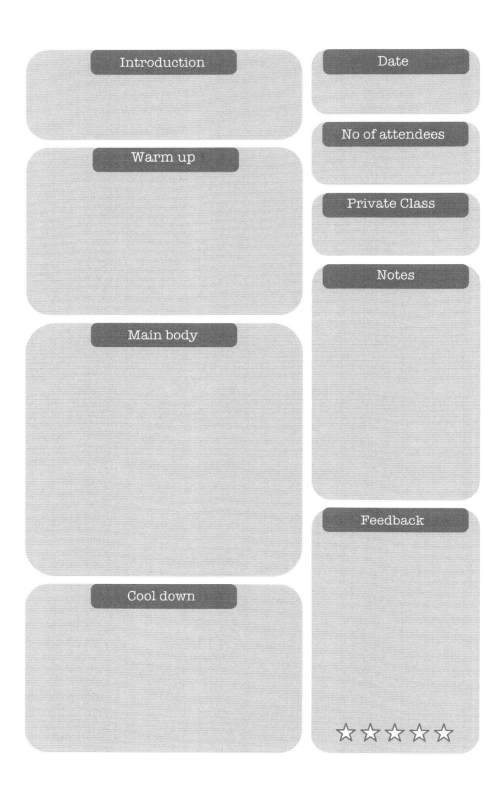

Introduction

Date

Warm up

No of attendees

Private Class

Main body

Notes

Feedback

Cool down

☆☆☆☆☆

Introduction

Warm up

Main body

Cool down

Date

No of attendees

Private Class

Notes

Feedback

☆☆☆☆☆

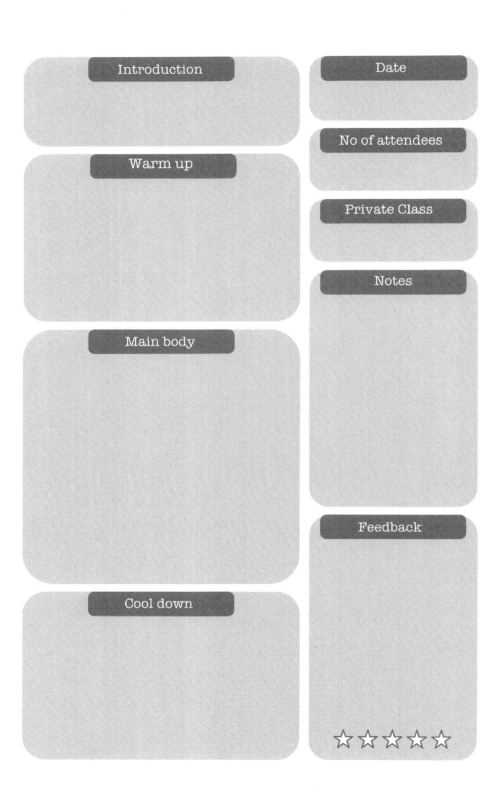

Introduction

Date

Warm up

No of attendees

Private Class

Main body

Notes

Cool down

Feedback

☆☆☆☆☆

Introduction

Date

No of attendees

Warm up

Private Class

Notes

Main body

Feedback

Cool down

★★★★☆

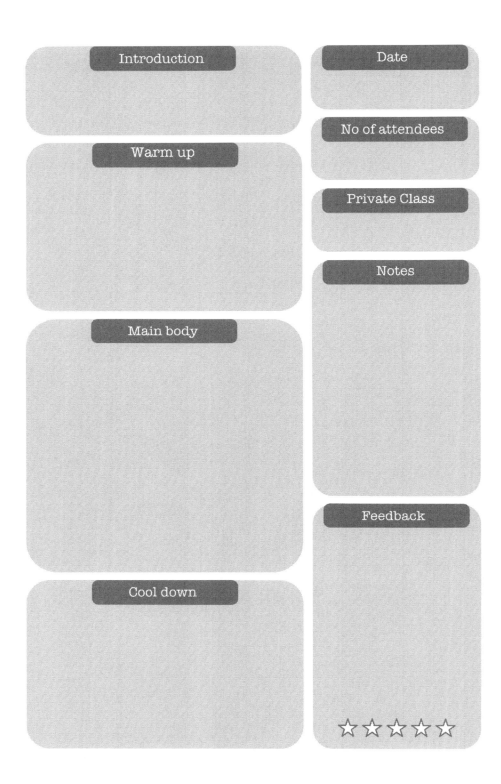

Introduction

Date

No of attendees

Warm up

Private Class

Notes

Main body

Cool down

Feedback

☆☆☆☆☆

Introduction

Warm up

Main body

Cool down

Date

No of attendees

Private Class

Notes

Feedback

☆ ☆ ☆ ☆ ☆

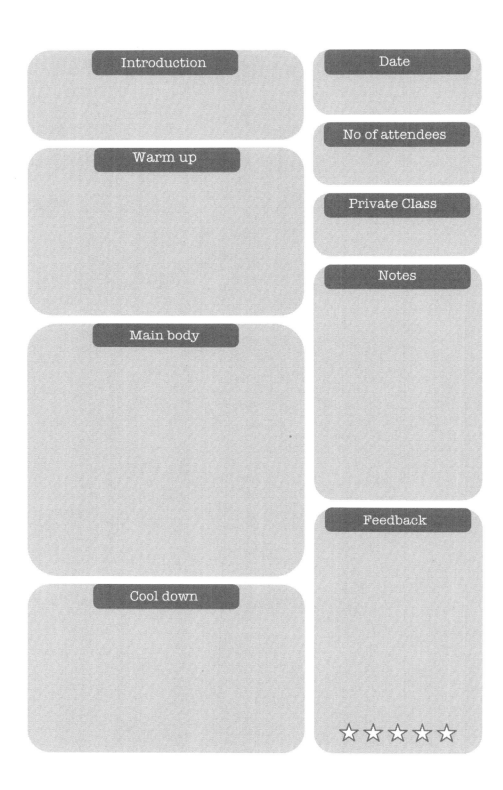

Introduction

Date

Warm up

No of attendees

Private Class

Notes

Main body

Cool down

Feedback

☆ ☆ ☆ ☆ ☆

Introduction

Date

Warm up

No of attendees

Private Class

Main body

Notes

Cool down

Feedback

☆☆☆☆☆

Introduction

Warm up

Main body

Cool down

Date

No of attendees

Private Class

Notes

Feedback

☆ ☆ ☆ ☆ ☆

Introduction

Date

No of attendees

Warm up

Private Class

Notes

Main body

Feedback

Cool down

☆ ☆ ☆ ☆ ☆

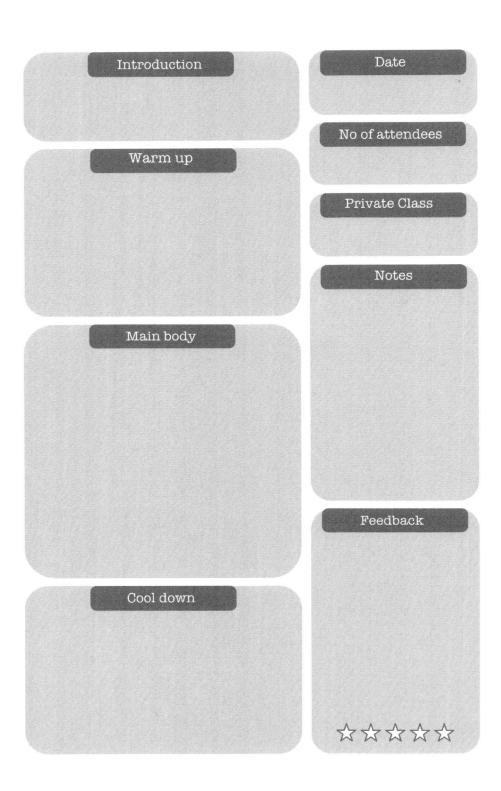

Introduction

Date

Warm up

No of attendees

Private Class

Main body

Notes

Cool down

Feedback

☆☆☆☆☆

Introduction

Date

No of attendees

Warm up

Private Class

Main body

Notes

Cool down

Feedback

☆ ☆ ☆ ☆ ☆

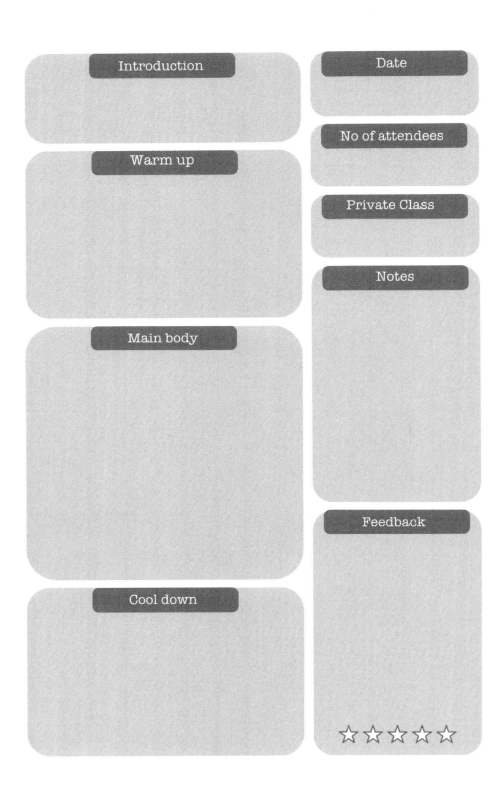

Introduction

Date

No of attendees

Warm up

Private Class

Notes

Main body

Cool down

Feedback

☆☆☆☆☆

Introduction

Date

Warm up

No of attendees

Private Class

Main body

Notes

Cool down

Feedback

☆☆☆☆☆

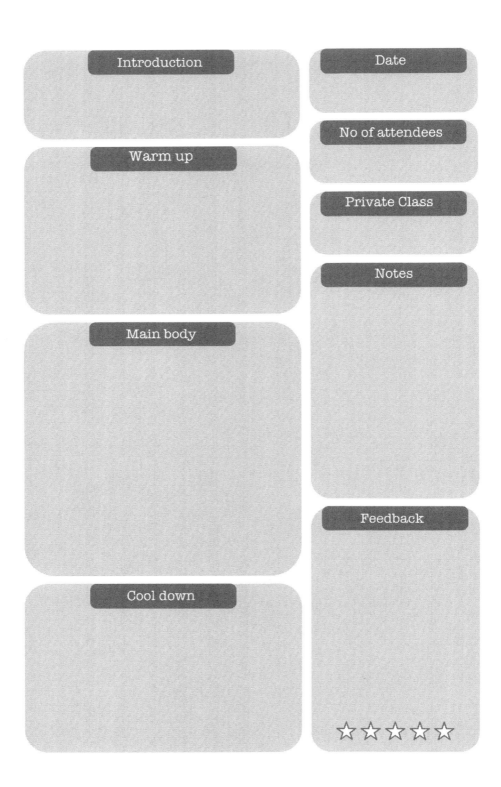

Introduction

Date

No of attendees

Warm up

Private Class

Notes

Main body

Feedback

Cool down

☆☆☆☆☆

Introduction

Date

No of attendees

Warm up

Private Class

Notes

Main body

Feedback

Cool down

☆ ☆ ☆ ☆ ☆

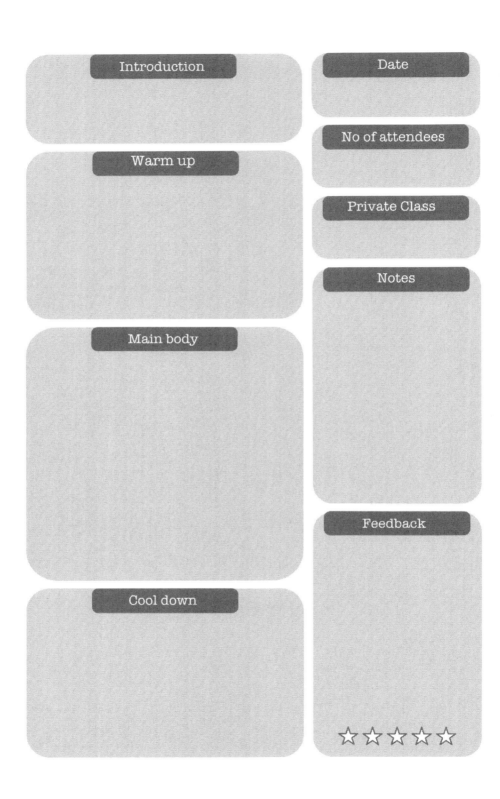

Introduction

Date

No of attendees

Warm up

Private Class

Notes

Main body

Feedback

Cool down

☆☆☆☆☆

Introduction

Date

No of attendees

Warm up

Private Class

Notes

Main body

Cool down

Feedback

☆☆☆☆☆

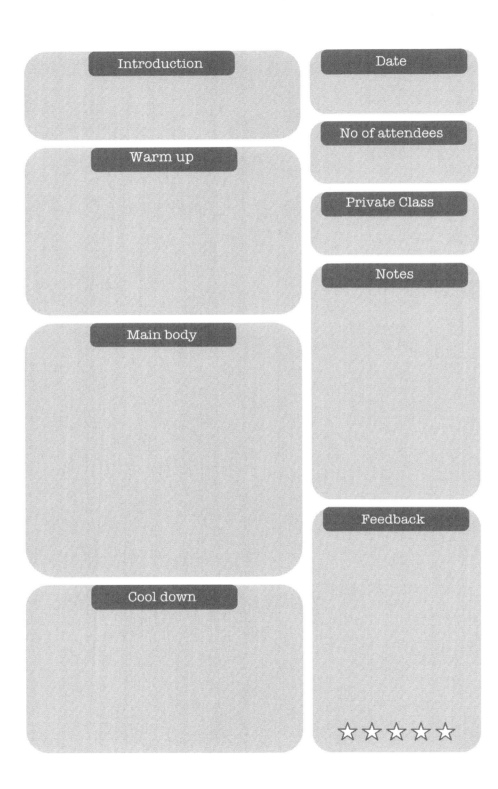

Introduction

Date

Warm up

No of attendees

Private Class

Main body

Notes

Feedback

Cool down

☆ ☆ ☆ ☆ ☆

Introduction

Date

Warm up

No of attendees

Private Class

Notes

Main body

Cool down

Feedback

☆☆☆☆☆

Introduction

Warm up

Main body

Cool down

Date

No of attendees

Private Class

Notes

Feedback

☆ ☆ ☆ ☆ ☆

Introduction

Date

Warm up

No of attendees

Private Class

Main body

Notes

Cool down

Feedback

☆☆☆☆☆

Introduction

Warm up

Main body

Cool down

Date

No of attendees

Private Class

Notes

Feedback

☆☆☆☆☆

Introduction

Date

No of attendees

Warm up

Private Class

Notes

Main body

Feedback

Cool down

☆ ☆ ☆ ☆ ☆

Introduction

Date

Warm up

No of attendees

Private Class

Notes

Main body

Feedback

Cool down

☆☆☆☆☆

Introduction

Warm up

Main body

Cool down

Date

No of attendees

Private Class

Notes

Feedback

☆☆☆☆☆

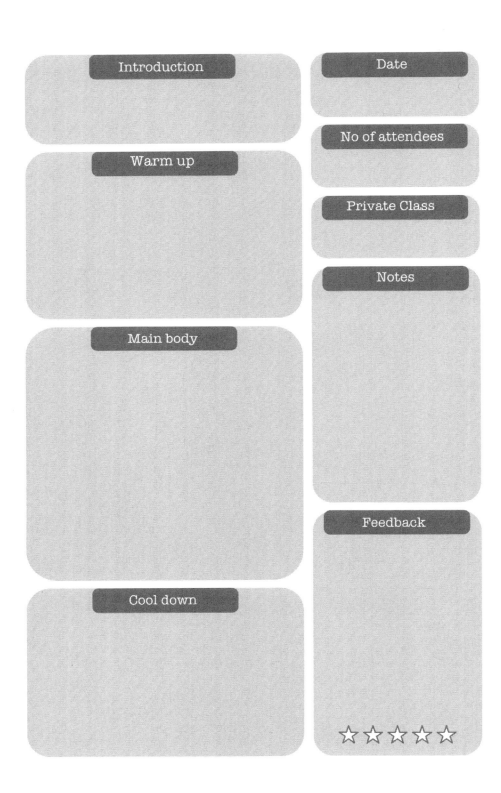

Introduction

Date

Warm up

No of attendees

Private Class

Main body

Notes

Feedback

Cool down

☆ ☆ ☆ ☆ ☆

Introduction

Date

No of attendees

Warm up

Private Class

Notes

Main body

Feedback

Cool down

☆☆☆☆☆

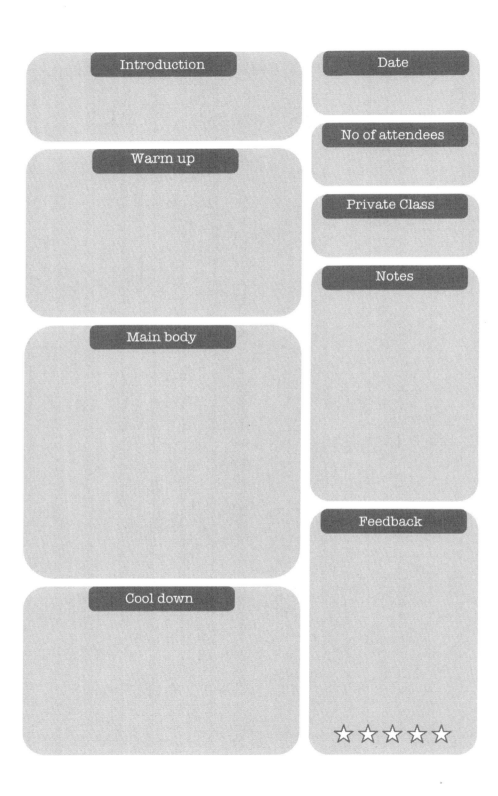

Introduction

Date

Warm up

No of attendees

Private Class

Main body

Notes

Feedback

Cool down

☆☆☆☆☆

Introduction

Date

Warm up

No of attendees

Private Class

Main body

Notes

Cool down

Feedback

☆ ☆ ☆ ☆ ☆

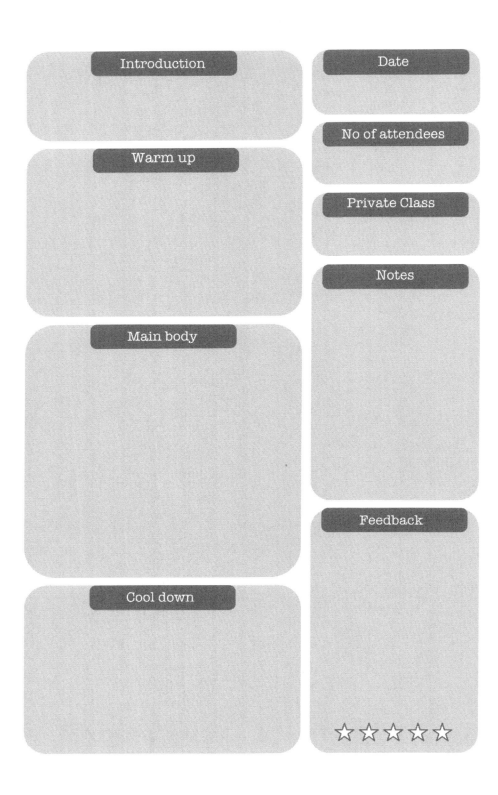

Introduction

Warm up

Main body

Cool down

Date

No of attendees

Private Class

Notes

Feedback

☆ ☆ ☆ ☆ ☆

Introduction

Warm up

Main body

Cool down

Date

No of attendees

Private Class

Notes

Feedback

☆☆☆☆☆

Introduction

Date

Warm up

No of attendees

Private Class

Notes

Main body

Cool down

Feedback

☆☆☆☆☆

Introduction

Date

Warm up

No of attendees

Private Class

Main body

Notes

Cool down

Feedback

☆ ☆ ☆ ☆ ☆

Introduction

Warm up

Main body

Cool down

Date

No of attendees

Private Class

Notes

Feedback

☆☆☆☆☆

Introduction

Date

No of attendees

Warm up

Private Class

Notes

Main body

Feedback

Cool down

☆ ☆ ☆ ☆ ☆

Introduction

Date

Warm up

No of attendees

Private Class

Main body

Notes

Cool down

Feedback

☆ ☆ ☆ ☆ ☆

Introduction

Date

Warm up

No of attendees

Private Class

Main body

Notes

Cool down

Feedback

☆ ☆ ☆ ☆ ☆

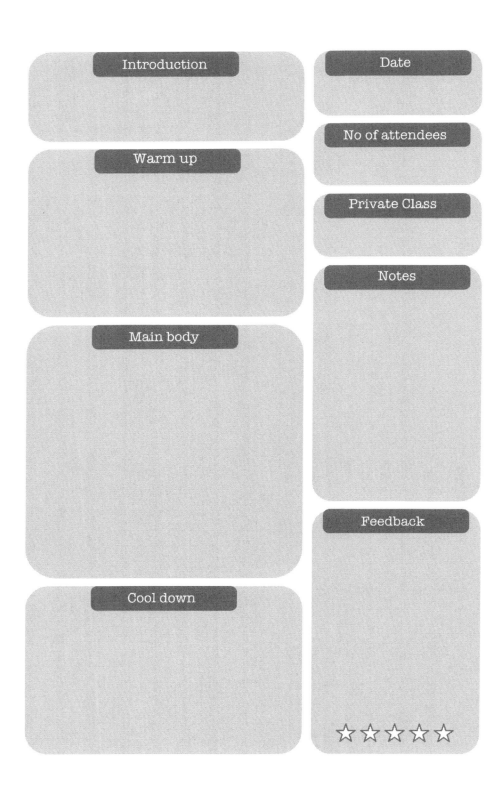

Introduction

Date

Warm up

No of attendees

Private Class

Notes

Main body

Feedback

Cool down

☆ ☆ ☆ ☆ ☆

Introduction

Date

Warm up

No of attendees

Private Class

Main body

Notes

Feedback

Cool down

☆ ☆ ☆ ☆ ☆

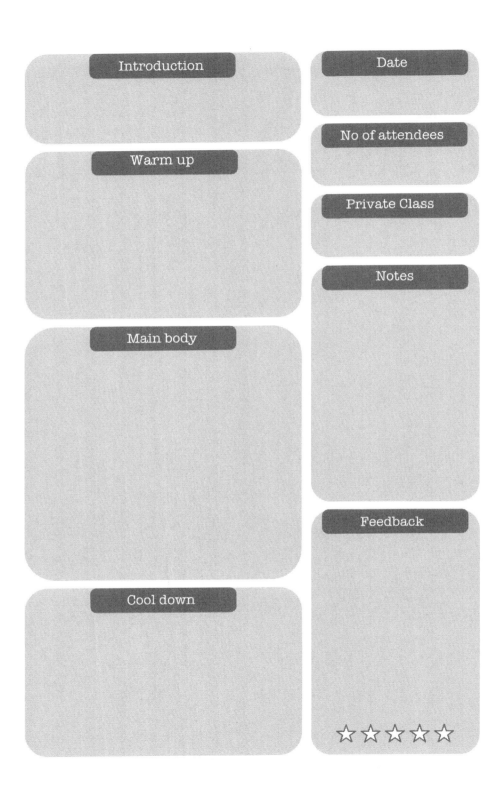

Introduction

Date

Warm up

No of attendees

Private Class

Notes

Main body

Feedback

Cool down

☆ ☆ ☆ ☆ ☆

Introduction

Date

Warm up

No of attendees

Private Class

Main body

Notes

Cool down

Feedback

☆☆☆☆☆

Introduction

Date

Warm up

No of attendees

Private Class

Main body

Notes

Cool down

Feedback

☆ ☆ ☆ ☆ ☆

Introduction

Warm up

Main body

Cool down

Date

No of attendees

Private Class

Notes

Feedback

☆ ☆ ☆ ☆ ☆

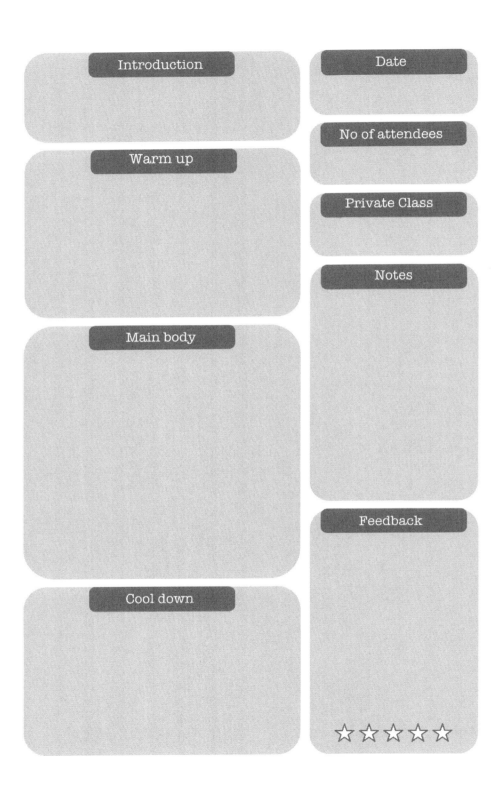

Introduction

Date

Warm up

No of attendees

Private Class

Main body

Notes

Cool down

Feedback

☆☆☆☆☆

Introduction

Date

No of attendees

Warm up

Private Class

Notes

Main body

Feedback

Cool down

☆ ☆ ☆ ☆ ☆

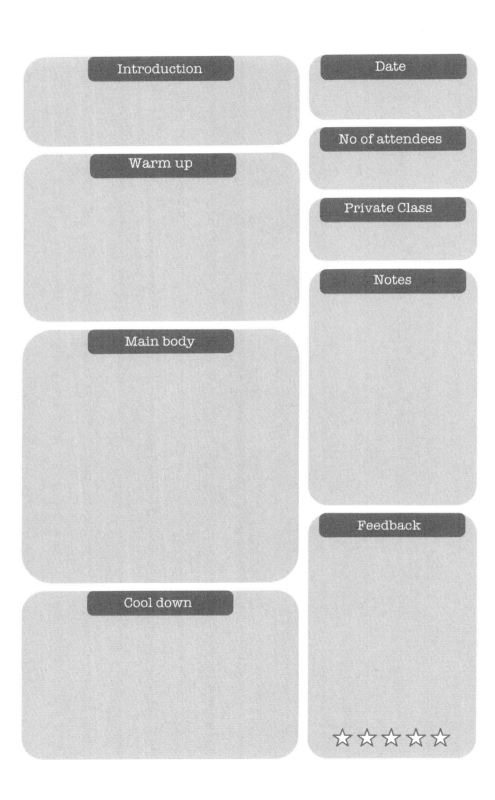

Introduction

Date

Warm up

No of attendees

Private Class

Notes

Main body

Cool down

Feedback

☆☆☆☆☆

Introduction

Warm up

Main body

Cool down

Date

No of attendees

Private Class

Notes

Feedback

☆ ☆ ☆ ☆ ☆

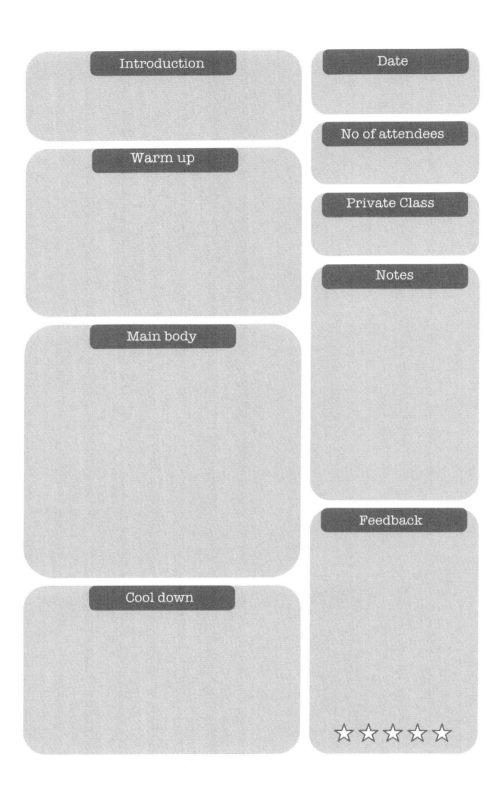

Introduction

Date

Warm up

No of attendees

Private Class

Main body

Notes

Feedback

Cool down

☆☆☆☆☆

Introduction

Date

Warm up

No of attendees

Private Class

Main body

Notes

Cool down

Feedback

☆☆☆☆☆

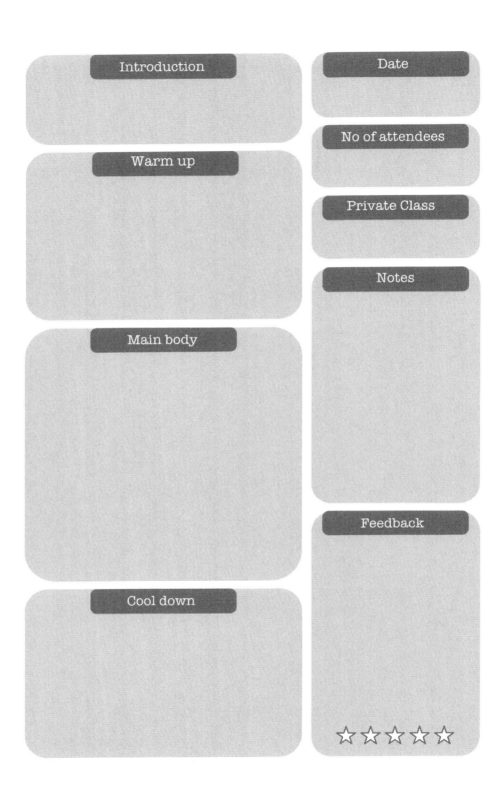

Introduction

Warm up

Main body

Cool down

Date

No of attendees

Private Class

Notes

Feedback

☆☆☆☆☆

Introduction

Date

No of attendees

Warm up

Private Class

Notes

Main body

Feedback

Cool down

☆ ☆ ☆ ☆ ☆

Introduction

Warm up

Main body

Cool down

Date

No of attendees

Private Class

Notes

Feedback

☆ ☆ ☆ ☆ ☆

Introduction

Warm up

Main body

Cool down

Date

No of attendees

Private Class

Notes

Feedback

☆ ☆ ☆ ☆ ☆

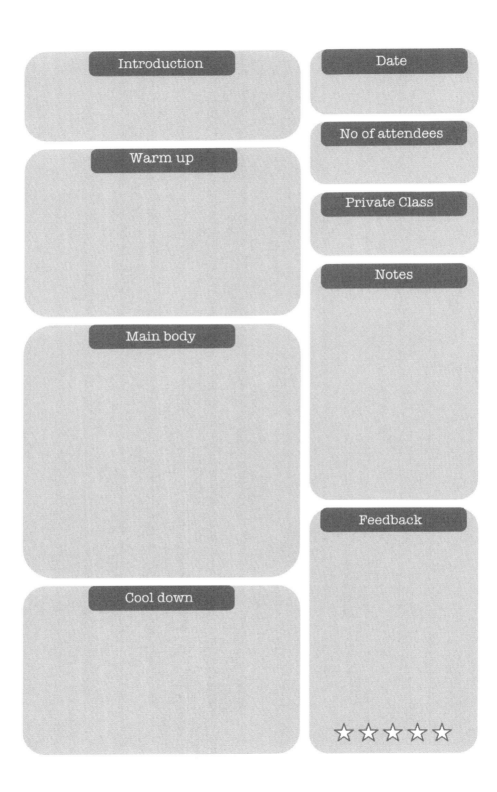

Introduction

Date

Warm up

No of attendees

Private Class

Main body

Notes

Feedback

Cool down

☆ ☆ ☆ ☆ ☆

Introduction

Date

Warm up

No of attendees

Private Class

Notes

Main body

Cool down

Feedback

☆ ☆ ☆ ☆ ☆

Introduction

Date

No of attendees

Warm up

Private Class

Main body

Notes

Feedback

Cool down

☆☆☆☆☆

Introduction

Date

No of attendees

Private Class

Warm up

Notes

Main body

Feedback

Cool down

☆☆☆☆☆

Notes

Printed in Great Britain
by Amazon